THE LITTLE BOOK OF POSITIVE THOUGHTS FOR CARERS

BRENDA MUNITICH

This book could not have been written without the loving support of my husband Fred and my children, Mark, Carolyn, Patricia, Diane and Robert.

PREFACE BY THE AUTHOR

Dear Carers,

Welcome to my world of caring. I have written this book based on my experiences over the past twenty years as a full time carer.

I have struggled through all the negative emotions described in the following pages. It wasn't until I found that by using the power of auto-suggestion, I could shift into positive thinking mode. It improved my life and the lives of the two people I care for far beyond our expectations. You could say we experienced a miracle!

I'm sure you will find positive thoughts between the pages of this little book that will work a miracle for you. After all, we do have a choice between negative and positive thinking.

Positive thinking opens the door to miracles!

Brenda Munitich

FORWARD

Carers are the most generous people we are ever likely to come across in our lives. Anyone who helps a friend or member of their family with practical and emotional support is a 'carer'. Carers, however, very rarely recognise the fact that they are carers and that they belong to this very special breed of people. They are unstinting in their love and never think twice in putting the person they care for first. Many carers give up work, education and leisure opportunities and often become socially isolated as the caring role becomes greater.

This book is an ideal *carer's handbook* to dip into when life throws up difficult times, when weariness sets in or when 'time out' is time limited. In many years of developing support services for carers, I cannot bring to mind a single carer I have met who would not benefit from picking up this little book and experiencing a few quiet reflective moments of *me time*.

The inspiration for this book has emanated from the author's own vast caring experiences and like most things in life, you can't beat first hand experience. So take on board Brenda's recommendations and remember your own health matters too. Look after yourself. As a carer myself, I plan to! And of course, enjoy the book!

Doris Dallimore

Manager, Bridgend Carers Centre

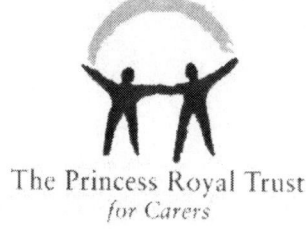

The Princess Royal Trust
for Carers

Contents

Resisting the changes in your circumstances is like trying to swim against the tide. Go with the flow and you will travel further.

ACCEPTANCE

Becoming a carer for your loved one or a family member at home will mean a change in your lifestyle and sacrificing part of your freedom.

Accept your position gracefully and determine to turn it into a life-enriching experience. There are valuable lessons to be learned from every situation no matter how difficult it may be. So how do you cope?

Start by looking for the strengths in you that you never knew you had, then concentrate on those strengths instead of your weaknesses.

Take responsibility for your thoughts from the beginning. Believe in yourself and prepare to cope with whatever happens. Acknowledge that you will be facing fresh challenges on the road ahead as your life takes a new direction. Don't focus on longing for the past, or any feelings of resentment about the situation you are now in.

There will be many people who will feel sympathy for you as they try to understand what it means to become a carer. Accept their sympathy. Their hearts are in the right place.

Make the most of each day and you will reap positive rewards.

ONE DAY AT A TIME

Starting each new day is like turning over the pages of a journal. The choice is yours to write the diary of your day. Ensure it will be a good day by counting your blessings when you wake up and thinking positive thoughts.

Yesterday is past, tomorrow becomes today, so make today your best possible day. *Now* is the only precious moment you have. Do your best, it adds to your future. Free yourself from the past and use the lessons you've learned to benefit you as a carer.

You may face a busy schedule and tasks that drain you physically, spiritually and mentally. Concentrate on one thing at a time and don't let your thoughts fly ahead so that you're doing one thing and coping with another, otherwise you will become confused and exhausted. Concentrate on the task in hand and live in the moment.

Every day set yourself small achievable goals that will add to the quality of your life. You will be amazed at the sense of achievement that you'll feel when you have reached the first goal. Your self-respect and confidence will soar. It's the little things that add up. The sea is made up of drops of water and what a mighty ocean it has become.

*Fear is our greatest enemy.
It weakens the foundations of
character.*

FEARS AND ANXIETIES

Of course you will be plagued by fears and anxieties, it is only natural. You'll have fears that something may go wrong with your loved one, anxiety about their welfare and whether or not you are coping well enough. These can be soul destroying emotions.

Fears are irrational because our imagination exaggerates and colours our thoughts. Fear closes a fist around your heart and causes negative vibrations that everyone around you will sense. Don't allow anxiety to diminish your self-confidence and capabilities.

What you think about you will attract into your life. Nothing outside of yourself can control you unless you allow it to. You are in control of your mind.

Banish your fears and anxieties with positive affirmations. "I am coping". "All is well". "There is nothing to fear except fear itself."

You are not a failure because you have anxious moments, everyone does. You are a success because you care about someone other than yourself. Be strong for them.

Make a list of positive affirmations and read inspirational books.

Give generously. The well of supply has an endless source.

GIVING

There's an old Chinese proverb that says 'If you desire a lifetime's happiness, help someone else.' What you sow, you will reap.

You will find happiness, not in self-indulgence, but by doing things for your loved ones. Love in action works miracles, both for you and for others. It is one of life's most powerful healing forces.

The most worthwhile giving is not in material gifts, but in giving positive words of encouragement, sincere compliments, friendship and happiness.

Smile, even when you are feeling low and you will be surprised at how smiling will give you and those around you a lift. Smiles are infectious; every feeling multiplies itself.

By bringing enjoyment into the lives of others, you will find happiness.

Your needs are important. Give yourself one or two small treats each day. It is not selfish or vain to look after your appearance. If you look good, you'll feel good; this will make you feel relaxed and enable you to give more of yourself to others around you.

In giving, your life will be enriched.

You are only lonely when you cease being friends with yourself.

LONELINESS

At times you may feel lonely and isolated from the rest of the world. You may feel as though people are avoiding you. They don't mean to; it's only because they are embarrassed and not sure how to approach someone with a physical disability or a mental illness.

Caring can be a lonely business. There are carers who prefer to be alone, who enjoy their own company. Many others crave company and feel the regular need to talk. Balance your day according to your needs. Make a plan to overcome loneliness if it is disquieting your peace of mind. Create your happiness according to your circumstances.

Don't compare yourself with other people who seem to have more freedom. Don't put yourself down when you are feeling tired and lonely. Reach out to at least one other person everyday, even if it's just a telephone call.

Ask someone to relieve you to give you a chance to go out for a few hours. Join a carers group. When talking with other carers you'll find that you are not alone in your feelings of loneliness, and this will make you feel better.

To be alone can also be a good thing. You can listen to the inner voice coming from your heart. When it speaks to you, you'll never be lonely.

Guilt stems from feelings of doubt, inadequacy and secrecy. Honest living makes a mockery of guilt.

GUILT

We can all experience guilty feelings from time-to-time for unkind thoughts we've had about other people. You may feel resentful about the situation you find yourself in and so feel guilty. If you allow these negative emotions to grow they will make you feel physically ill.

When you think thoughts of love towards the person you have wrongly judged, your guilt will slowly disappear. There is always something to love in everyone, even in the most difficult of circumstances.

Forgive yourself when you make mistakes and don't feel guilty about them. Life is not perfect, neither are human beings. If you judge yourself harshly it will be difficult for you to be kind to others.

Banish the phrase "I should" from your vocabulary and replace it with "I could". The word *should* is associated with procrastination and that fuels guilt.

Develop the capacity to understand your loved one's point of view. At the same time learn to say "No" to unreasonable requests.

Positive visualization and loving affirmations will help you grow as a person and dispel any feelings of guilt you may have experienced as a carer.

Endure while you can.
Time changes everything.

ENDURANCE

There may well be times when you feel downhearted, when you can see no end to your struggles. It needs courage to endure what can seem like an impossible situation; complaining or giving in has never solved a problem.

If you endure and persist, you will eventually win through and become a stronger person. Never give in to negative moments for that is all they are – passing moments.

Through your positive actions, determination and fortitude, you will pass on to those around you, your ability to endure difficult times. You will find new ways to succeed and will feel a renewed enthusiasm for life because you know you have the endurance to see you through dark and trying days.

Endurance means, faith, self-control and discipline.

Love what you are doing for your loved ones. Loving thoughts have healing vibrations.

Through coping with having to endure trying times, you will begin to feel a new respect for yourself.

Never, ever give up!

Resentment wears a cloak of nettles.

RESENTMENT

"Why me?" you may ask when you are feeling depressed and exhausted. "I didn't ask to become a carer. I feel trapped and lonely most days. No one calls around anymore because they feel they might be a nuisance."

Resentment destroys friendships. There's no point in moaning about your circumstances because no one will want to listen to you. People will avoid you.

Self-pity laced with resentment is one of the most destructive emotions I know of. It lowers your self-esteem and your self image. Use the positive aspects of caring to build you up instead of allowing it to undermine you.

Throw self-pity out of the window. Make a determined stand to change your attitude. Be proud that you have been chosen to be a carer because you are good enough to be one.

Take stock of yourself and ask yourself these questions. "If someone had to change places with me and take care of me would I want them to feel resentful and sorry for themselves?" Of course you wouldn't.

Stand back and take a long hard look at your situation. Is it so bad? Could it be worse?

Some people criticise to make themselves feel superior.

Those who criticise others are reflecting their own shortcomings.

CRITICISM

Criticism nourishes the seed of discontent that leads to unhappiness, whilst doing nothing to solve the problem.

Do you feel that others are criticising you by suggesting "Why don't you do this…?" or "You should do that." Don't take this to heart. Perhaps they want to be helpful…but how many would willingly change places with you?

Do you react to people and events by labelling and categorizing them? Are you finding fault with your circumstances or your loved one? Stop and think of the harm you are doing to them and to yourself.

Criticism undermines relationships and friendships.

Look for something good in everyone. Look for the blessings in your situation instead of criticising those who are trying to help you.

A sharp tongue indicates discontent within the person who is handing out criticisms and leads to their thoughts becoming warped. Always wanting to be right makes others wrong. A secure and happy person will always look for the best in other people.

Try going through a day without passing judgement on yourself or others. You'll feel less tense and much happier.

Exhaustion happens when you stop listening to your body.

DEALING WITH EXHAUSTION

There are times when you'll feel stretched beyond your limits and you'll ask yourself "Is it worth struggling on?"

When you are physically and mentally exhausted, negative factors in your life tend to become exaggerated to the point where they can overwhelm you. Problems manifest where no problems existed before and you become depressed when everything seems too much for you to handle. Your thoughts become confused and you forget things. You feel trapped in despair. "Stop the world," you cry, "I want to get off!"

Don't blame others for the way you are feeling. There is only one person who can help you and that is yourself.

The struggling ends when you stop thinking of it as a struggle.

Sit down, close you eyes, take a deep breath and slowly exhale counting down from eight to one. Picture yourself stepping down into a beautiful garden of sweet scented flowers. Listen to the birds singing and stroll across a bridge over a murmuring stream. When you open your eyes you will feel refreshed. Gaze up at the night sky with its moon and glittering stars and drink deeply from the beauty of nature. You will no longer feel so exhausted. Beautiful thoughts produce healing results.

Plant tiny seeds of positive thoughts in your mind and before long your life will bloom like a beautiful garden.

AUTO-SUGGESTION

All the resources you need as a carer are in your mind.

Such is the power of your thoughts that through the medium of auto-suggestion you can see a situation as being either negative or positive. Tell yourself you're tired and you'll feel tired.

Success can be measured by the way you handle your daily life and how well you communicate with other people. Reflect on the things you are good at. It's the small daily achievements that count; they all originate from auto-suggestion. Become the change you wish to see.

Think you are a failure and you will be. Think you are successful and you will attract success into your life. By success I don't mean that you will necessarily become wealthy overnight, but step by step, you will notice how life flows so much more effortlessly with positive thoughts.

Remind yourself that you are unique, that you are a caring person and that you are coping well. Carers are special.

Ease your aches and pains through auto-suggestion. Smiling is an uplifting remedy. Your body responds to the feel good factor of a smile. Think happy thoughts and you will begin to feel happier.

Banish procrastination from your life through the power of your thinking. Dare to be positive; when you begin you are already halfway there.

To pour your heart out through the medium of a pen is as relaxing as a tranquilliser.

KEEP A JOURNAL

A journal is a carer's best friend. Keep it close to your heart.

In a journal you can express your feelings in complete privacy, without fear of judgement or of upsetting anyone. You can *scream* through the written word and no one will ever hear.

A journal is an outlet for your emotions and on a more positive note, for listing your daily achievements.

After a while of disciplining yourself to write daily, you'll no longer need discipline; instead you will look forward to picking up a pen and writing about your day.

If you're too tired to write at night, then write in the early morning before anyone else is awake. A few minutes to write a few lines are all you need.

Keeping a five year journal is fun. You can look back over the years and keep track of your positive progress, your health and your daily activities.

A journal never betrays you, it never criticises, and it's never moody.

Shakespeare wrote "The pen is mightier than the sword."

Cheerful patience is the sign of a wise and gentle carer.

PATIENCE

Carers need patience – great dollops of it. The person you are caring for can be demanding, quarrelsome and critical. It's not their fault that they're feeling ill and at odds with themselves, you and the rest of the world.

Accept the fact that sometimes life must unfold in its own time. Impatience destroys the quality of your life and your relationships.

Your face reflects your emotions. Impatience and irritability will leave you feeling tense and strained; this will show in your face, leaving you looking tired and older. If you are impatient and rush around, you're more likely to misjudge events and make mistakes.

Be patient with yourself when you're feeling stressed or agitated. Take a few deep breaths. Patience calms your mind and thoughts.

With patience, your perceptions will sharpen and you will become more aware of your own needs. Allow the universe to take care of your needs. If you trust, listen and wait, all will fall into place at the right time; this will add to the quality of your life.

Patience is being active. It is an act of waiting without agitation or complaint.

To listen to another person is a sign of good manners.

To listen to your own body's needs is a necessity.

LISTEN

Listen to your needs.

You are only human and it's up to you to discipline yourself. How can you be disciplined if you don't listen to your intuition and your body's needs?

If your body tells you it needs a rest – obey it – even if it is just for a ten minute *power-nap*.

If your intuition tells you something, then listen to it; it is never wrong.

Once you understand yourself, you can make a point of trying to understand others. By listening, you learn so much about other people and a great deal about yourself too.

Carers need to talk and share their experiences. Listen to what other carers have to say and share your feelings with them. Talking helps to put things in to perspective.

Create harmony in your situation by listening to the person you are caring for. Respect their point of view; talking may be their only form of release.

Listen without judgement, interruption or pushing forward your point of view. Try to step into the mind of the person speaking to fully understand their perspective. Your loved one will be happier and this will make life easier for both of you.

To forgive and forget is the best plan for a peaceful existence.

FORGIVENESS

Forgiveness needs courage and strength; the rewards will be far beyond your expectations. You will feel as though a burden has been lifted from you when you say "I forgive you."

Forgive yourself for your mistakes and the things you wish you'd never said. Brooding over mistakes will cloud your perceptions and hold you back from making the most of your life.

Judging others harshly and harbouring thoughts of resentment, revenge, anger or hate will make you a prisoner of your feelings, causing emotional pain to you and others. The tension that results from such negative thoughts could leave you feeling physically ill and weakened.

Until you break the chains of negative and destructive thoughts, replacing them with positive affirmations of forgiveness, you will remain feeling like a prisoner.

Forgiveness means learning compassion and understanding.

If you forgive others you will reap forgiveness for things you may have said or done to upset someone. As you give, so you receive.

Forgiveness needs courage and generosity.

Forgiveness is an act of love.

If you are looking for the secret to success, look within yourself.

LETTING GO

Letting go is another way of accepting people and situations as they are. Letting go means we no longer judge or try to control others. It is immensely liberating and frees you from feeling stressed.

It isn't always easy to 'let go' of habits. A desire to be in control gives you a false sense of security. Being judgemental gives you an illusory idea of superiority and self-righteousness. Let go of your critical attitude and look for the good in everyone and everything.

There are times when we set high standards for ourselves and then feel like a failure when we don't achieve what we set out to do. Let go of such feelings of failure and use them instead as a learning experience.

Let go of relationships that create a feeling of obligation. "I should contact so and so," or "I should do this or that for them." A good relationship flows when communication between you is easy without pretence or obligation.

Let go of friendships with people who try to impress you with their wealth or social standing. True value lies in setting your own standards and not being swayed by others.

Allow your life to take its course by 'letting go.'

NOW is the most important moment in your life.

LIVING IN THE MOMENT

Stop, take a deep breath and savour this moment.

Pay attention to your thoughts. Are they flitting, like a butterfly, from one subject to another? Are you churning up the past and worrying about the future, so preoccupied with planning ahead that you miss out on the value of the present moment?

At times we are so busy rushing around that we skim the surface of life without taking time to appreciate the deeper meaning of things. We miss out on getting to know people well enough to form lasting friendships. Do you listen to others without hearing what they are saying because you are so busy thinking about putting over your point of view?

While eating, are you always in too much of a hurry to taste and appreciate your food?

You were lucky to be chosen to be born and to be who you are. You are unique. Be grateful for every moment that you are alive.

If you cultivate the habit of living fully in each moment, your life will be enriched beyond your expectations. You will feel more, hear more, see more, and become more sensitive to your needs.

Change is the enemy of boredom.

CHANGE

Change is as necessary for your well-being as food and water. Don't allow yourself to be drawn into a boring routine that leaves you feeling exhausted and fed-up. What you need is a significant change and variety and the freedom to do as you please at least once a week.

You don't have to leave your home to make changes that will leave you feeling refreshed. Start with small changes in your daily routine. Try out a new recipe, or even re-arrange your furniture.

On a more personal level try, wearing a different colour, one that suits you and makes you feel good. Ladies, try a different hairstyle or some new make-up.

As a busy carer you might not find it easy to take a holiday. Instead, indulge in an imaginary holiday in sunny surroundings. Find ten minutes, sit back, close your eyes and travel to your favourite places. Before long you'll experience the sensations of being there, such as the smell the sea, warm sunshine, a breeze on your face...

Listen to different music or read a different author. This way your mind will never grow stale, numbed by routine.

Don't let the fire go out of your life. The small changes you make will benefit both you and your loved one.

Live with the right colours around you. It brings magic into your life.

COLOURS

Few of us realise how much colour dominates our lives.

We need to live with the colours that are right for us because we respond to them.

Colour has a great impact on our minds, bodies and spirits. It stimulates, heals or calms us. Wearing colours that suit you will increase your self-esteem.

Green represents an affinity and oneness with nature, and is considered to bring you luck, while red restores vitality. Yellow is invigorating and uplifting. Blue has a magic all of its own. Think of blue skies, bluebells and forget-me-nots.

Orange is a happy colour; it stimulates the mind and lifts the spirits. Indigo is spiritual, meditative, and inspirational while brown is nurturing and supportive.

Fill your vases with brightly coloured flowers; they are good for your soul and for your loved one too.

Our appetites are stimulated by the colours of the food we eat. Arrange vegetables and fruits on your plates to tempt your appetites.

Become aware of colour and use its magic to improve your health and vitality in order to lead a better quality of life.

To be at peace with yourself is the greatest happiness.

HAPPINESS

Ella Wheeler Wilcox wrote "Laugh and the world laughs with you." Ponder on the wisdom of her words.

We all need to laugh. If you can be a happy personality and make people laugh or smile you will never be short of friends. Learning to cultivate a sense of humour will tide you over any difficult times.

There are two sides to everything in life depending on which way you see things. When possible, try to see the funny side.

Laughter or even a smile will release tensions in you which would otherwise restrict the sense of fun in being alive. *Smile* when you talk, allowing it to reach your eyes. Happiness is both therapeutic and cathartic.

A sense of humour unites young and old, the sick and the healthy; it helps to create a happy atmosphere.

Don't rely on external circumstances for your happiness. Forget about self-pity or resentment; instead look within yourself for happiness, because it is *always* a possibility that you can choose.

Make the choice to think pleasant thoughts and be grateful for the blessings and love that surround you.

Smile and soon your world will be smiling with you.

Life can be cold and lonely if you take away the warmth of friendship.

KEEPING IN TOUCH

"No man is an island unto himself," wrote John Donne. We all need people even if we like to think of ourselves as loners. Caring can create a solitary environment for you and your loved one. You may find at times that you feel agitated with each other, becoming bad tempered and over-reacting to situations.

It is important to keep in touch with other people otherwise you can grow in on yourself and become full of self pity, which breeds discontent. Don't allow your emotions to drain away until you feel cold and empty. You need to talk and unburden your feelings to someone who will listen.

Keep in touch with other people if you are housebound. All it takes is a telephone call, a note by post, or even an email to invite someone in for coffee and a chat. Find time to go shopping or join your local library.

It is important to join a support group where you will meet other carers. There are always professional people who will be happy to give you advice if you are becoming mentally or emotionally stressed and feel that you are no longer able to cope.

Don't be afraid to reach out. You are not alone.

Learn to love yourself.

All things on this earth are ruled by the miracles of nature.

LEARN FROM NATURE

Become aware of nature, of its natural rhythms and beauty. Nature takes its own course and never hurries. In nature there is harmony, healing and soothing beauty in the changing seasons.

When you lose touch with nature your spirit is starved of magic. Walk barefoot and feel the earth beneath your feet; feel the wind in your hair. Imagine you are walking along a beach, feel the sand soft and warm beneath your toes and the sea spray on your face.

Take a walk down a leafy lane. Cross a stream over stepping stones and look down into the sparkling, running water. Feed birds in your garden and listen to their songs of thanks.

Breathe in the smell of freshly mown grass or wet earth, the fragrance of roses or lavender. If you don't have a garden, or much time to work in a garden, grow flowers in pots, or herbs on your kitchen window sill. Watching them grow and mature will give you a sense of inner satisfaction, and touch your soul. There's a modern saying, "A garden grows people as well as plants."

Flowers are a token of friendship, love and peace.

Flowers are nature's perfection.

You need time and space for yourself to rediscover your identity.

TIME FOR YOURSELF

Look down on your life as though you were seeing it from above. How do you see yourself? Can you find yourself, or has your identity been submerged in the rush of the day's activities?

You need to make time and space, even half an hour a day, to keep in touch with your inner self. Find somewhere quiet in your bedroom or your garden where you can sit without interruption from anyone, and think about yourself and your needs.

Let all burdens fall from your shoulders. In a relaxed and calm manner, remind yourself that as a carer, all things are working together for your good and that you are a tower of strength.

You have a right to physical health. The best exercises, walking and deep breathing, are free and you don't need to go far from your home.

Take up a hobby, a creative activity that you enjoy and choose one that you can share with a friend if you wish to. It is an insurance against the boredom of routine and takes your mind off any immediate problems. Listen to music or read a good book.

Reward yourself with "me" time. You deserve it.

We are a reflection of our thoughts, words and deeds.

REFLECTIONS

Reflect on your life, past and present, your weaknesses and your strengths. Ask yourself questions and answer them truthfully. If you cannot be honest with yourself then who can you be honest with?

Do I like myself? Am I doing my best for my loved one and making the most of my situation? Do I feel guilty about something that's not my fault? Reflect on your answers to these questions.

Take a good look at your habits. Habits are the repetition of actions that make you the person you are. Your habits live with you and become part of your identity. Don't allow bad habits to shadow your life. Make a list of the bad habits you want to break then replace them with good ones.

Good habits mean a repetition of positive words like, "I can...." They also include your health, your eating, your thinking and your daily living.

Make it a habit to use positive words. Your subconscious registers with your habitual thinking, so it becomes your identity and your destiny.

Take back control of your destiny by visualizing the things you want to come true in your life.

Silence opens the way for meditation.

MEDITATION

Meditation is the practice of mindfulness in a silence that allows you to listen to the voice of your intuition. The more you practice meditation the more it will allow your instincts to guide you.

Meditation reduces stress; it is calming and comforting and it puts you in touch with your inner self.

You need time alone to meditate. When you are a full time carer it is not always easy to find the time. Try waking up half an hour earlier when your household is quiet; noise drains your energy.

To meditate properly you need to sit or lie in a comfortable position, close your eyes, silence your thoughts and empty your mind. Breathe deeply in and out, relaxing every muscle in your body while you concentrate on your breathing.

Your thoughts may dart here and there at first, but with practise, you can learn to control and discipline your thinking. Ask your subconscious to guide you and it will. Listen to and follow your instincts; they are never wrong. You will feel less stressed and more at peace with your situation.

Meditation teaches you to love yourself. When you love yourself you have more love to give to others.

To be born is a miracle.

BELIEVE IN YOURSELF

Life is a miracle. That you were chosen to be born is a miracle.

That your loved one has you to care for him or her is a miracle because you are the best carer for them.

Never stop believing that your loved one's condition will improve or be healed because belief is the magic word that creates miracles. The medical world is making rapid strides towards finding cures for many illnesses, physical and mental.

A miracle doesn't have to be a big explosive happening that sets bells ringing; it more often comes in the form of little day to day happenings.

Never stop visualizing and believing in your hopes and dreams. They are miracles waiting to happen.

If you look out and beyond your world, you will appreciate the way that nature performs miracles with its changing seasons to provide us with the food we need to for our survival.

Count your blessings, believe more will come and they will.

Your blessings are a miracle.

Music is a medium for healing, peace and harmony.

THE INSPIRATION OF MUSIC

Music lifts depression and awakens your inner consciousness.

Harmonious vibration from music inspires love, good health, peace and heals your soul. The sounds of soothing music can also be beneficial and relaxing for your loved one.

If you feel lonely, listen to music that really inspires and uplifts you as a background for your thoughts. Music can create positive thoughts and re-connect you with pleasant memories.

Have you ever stopped to listen to a bird singing, its notes pure and joyful? It touches your soul.

Music stirs your emotions and raises your spirits. It can bring you to tears – there is no harm in shedding a few tears to release tension.

Music is food for the soul and brings with it kind and loving thoughts. So make it a habit to include some music in your routine to lighten your role as a carer.

ACKNOWLEDGEMENTS

My sincere thanks to my daughter, Diane MacDowall and her partner, Andrew Nicholson for their unwavering encouragement and for editing my book to a publishable standard.

The Little Book of Positive Thoughts for Carers

AUTHOR PROFILE

This "Little Book of Positive Thoughts for Carers" has been written by a woman who has been a carer for most of her life. As a teenager, eldest of seven children, she helped her mother to raise her six siblings.

Brenda Munitich lives in Bridgend, South Wales where she cares for her husband and son. She is the mother of five children, six grandchildren and a great-grandson.

She has always been an ardent believer in the power of positive thinking, applying it to her daily living.

As a full time carer she still manages to write, enjoy life and inspire others. She finds *me time* and uses positive thinking to fill her soul with enough self-love so that she can spill it over in abundance to those she cares for.

Lightning Source UK Ltd.
Milton Keynes UK
06 January 2011
165265UK00002B/248/P